Art of Breathing

for

Stress Free Life

By Subodh Gupta
Corporate Yoga Trainer

First Edition September 2007

ISBN 978-1-84799-047-1

Library of Congress Control Number: 2007907962

Published by
Subodh Gupta
Head office: London (UK)
Email: info@subodhgupta.com
Website: www.subodhgupta.com
44(0)7966275913

Publisher Note:
The reader should not regard the recommendation and breathing techniques expressed and described in this book as substitute advice of a qualified medical practitioner. It is also advisable that reader may learn the breathing exercises initially in the presence of qualified yoga trainer.

Acknowledgements

I am grateful to all my teachers who taught me at various stages of my life & shared with me their wisdom.

Content

Introduction 6

Part 1:

Understanding about breath 9

Type of breath 12

Why the speech of CEO & leaders is thrilling 17

Part 2:

Technique 1: Deep Breathing Exercise 23

Technique 2: Full Yogic Breathing 25

Technique 3: Kapalabhati Exercise 27

Technique 4: Alternate Nostril breathing (Without Breath retention) 33

Technique 5: Alternate Nostril Breathing (With Breath Retention) 39

Stress Monitor 47

Practice Record 48

Introduction:

Imagine you are getting ready for board meeting or presentation feeling tense and you knew the art of relaxing your mind within minutes!!!

Imagine you can stay energetic and full of energy throughout the day. Imagine that you have the skill to establish yourself in state of tranquillity anytime. Of course it may seem like magic trick but reality is, people who are aware and adept in yogic breathing exercises can easily do it.

You can do it too, because breathing is one physical function which is both involuntary (going by itself) and voluntary (it can be control consciously).

Effective breathing is very important and essential for good health. If you find yourself getting tired easily or stressed, you can improve the situation by breathing exercises and you would be amazed to see how quickly you can improve your stamina and reduce your stress.

This simple and significant insight into art of breathing was known to scientists of India (discovering inner dimension of human being) thousands of years ago.

This knowledge and technique of Yogic breathing is explained in this book in a step by step method along with precautions in simplest possible way so that everybody can understand and gain benefit.

This book has been divided into 2 sections.

Section 1 contains knowledge and explanation of breath from various perspectives and section 2 includes five practical techniques step by step. It is important to read section 1 first before trying simple breathing techniques.

In the end, I have provided tools for self assessing stress and tracking your progress. It is a good idea to fill these sheets after practicing everyday breathing techniques to identify the difference over a period of 4 weeks. Please remember that everyday practice is must otherwise all theory and no practice would not lead you anywhere.

If you are practicing everyday in a correct way then positive results will certainly be there.

After the breathing exercises you would definitely feel relaxed and calm. If you feel tired or uncomfortable in that case you need to check if you are practicing in wrong way.

I wish all of you who read this book to get the maximum benefit in terms of achieving radiant health and stress free life.

May everybody be Stress free and Peaceful.

Subodh Gupta

"Flow of breath can give clear picture about person emotional and mental state"

Part 1:

Understanding about Breath

You will agree with me that since the time you came on this planet earth (the time you were born) and till now as you are reading this book, you are constantly breathing without interruption. So let me ask you one basic question. How many times do you breathe in a day??? (One breath equals to one inhalation and one exhalation).

..

..

..

..

..

Any idea or guess, still thinking ....

Ok, let me give you the answer.

We usually take about 13-15 breaths in a minute. This way if you count, the total numbers of breaths comes to 18720 - 21,600 times per day or say around 20000 times in a day.

Yes, you are reading correctly around twenty thousand times in a day. Now you might be thinking that why I am asking you such kind of question. The reason is I want to emphasise the fact that breathing is one of the most important function in our body but it is most neglected one. It influences the activity of each and every cell in our body and most importantly it is intimately linked with the performance of the brain.

Breath is the life force that sustains life. When the breath stops, life ends. Simple breathing exercise helps to control this life force in an extraordinary way to get the tremendous benefits. It brings benefits such as increased energy and perception, and development of various brain faculties.

Normally most people use only a fraction of their lungs capacity for breathing. The breathing which is shallow deprives the body of oxygen and energy and it leads to disharmony in the body. This results in hunched shoulders. Many people get tired easily in their daily working schedule and do not realize why? This could be corrected by proper breathing exercise. With simple deep and controlled breathing exercises the absorption of energy can be increased, which enhances dynamism and general wellbeing. Awareness and control of the breath also allows us to control our emotions. So proper breathing is must and required for maintaining good health and liveliness.

Why it is important to develop the awareness of breath and gain conscious control over it?

Our body cannot live without life energy/breath and if breath is allowed to run on its own, then our unconscious mind controls our breath and the breath is effected (you can notice it when you start observing yourself).

Whenever our state of mind is disturbed then our breath is also disturbed for long time and it is not good for the health in long run.

However, if we are aware of our breath, we can be aware of our mental state. By learning few breathing techniques we can consciously control our breath and can even manage our mental and emotional state rather than to be controlled by it.

Link of Breath, mind and body

Breath is the link between body and mind. Breath can be regulated by the mind or it can be left to the body. Although breath is not controlled by either of them exclusively but can be effected by both of them and in turn affect both of them and is the key to the interaction of body and mind.

Breath and Emotions:

There is a direct relationship between the breath of a person and his / her emotional state. Flow of breath can give clear picture about a person emotional and mental state. When the breath is relaxed and slow it gives an indication of calmness however, if the breath is uneven and disrupted it gives an indication of emotional and mental disturbance. Breath can be agitated if the person is angry, it can be stopped momentarily in case of fear, it can be choked in sadness and sighing with relief etc. Physical exercise can change the emotional state of person and so does his/ her breath.

Emotional and mental state of person are difficult to control however they are linked with breath and breath can be controlled, i.e. emotional and mental state of human being can also be controlled by controlling breath. In day to day life normally people use following four types of breathing.

Type of Breath

For simplicity of the readers, I have avoided going much into technical terminology of breathing and have chosen breath pattern from practical point of view which everybody can easily understand. There are 4 different ways which people use for breathing in their day to day life.

(a) Clavicular breathing

(b) Thoracic Breathing / Chest Breathing

(c) Paradoxical Breathing

(d) Deep Abdominal Breathing / Diaphragmatic breathing

Clavicular breathing is the most shallow and least effective breathing. Its name derives from the two clavicles or you can say two collarbones, which are pulled upwards when you complete your inhalation. In this breathing shoulders and collarbone area are raised and abdomen is contracted during inhaling the breath. In this type of breathing one has to apply the maximum effort to breathe in and minimum amount of air is inhaled. We get very little energy from atmosphere in this type of breath. In day to day life clavicular breathing is rarely used except under extreme conditions when body's energy demand is great during extreme physical exertion.

Thoracic breathing or Chest Breathing is done with rib muscles expanding the rib cage. This breathing is usually shallow and rapid. This breathing technique fills the middle and upper portion of lungs with air however it is not good enough for the lower portion. If you are in standing position, most of the blood would be in lower area of lungs because of the gravity so the gas exchange which takes place between air in the lungs and blood would not be complete.

This is the type of breathing which is often associated with physical exercise and stress/ tension. I have seen mostly in gym people are using this breathing technique however people continue this kind of breathing even after they come out of gym which results into unhealthy breathing habit.

This breathing is better than clavicular but not complete as well because the amount of air inhaled is less as compare to deep abdominal breathing. Also it results in more work for the heart as compared to diaphragmatic breathing because chest breathing requires comparatively more work for blood and gases mixing, so more oxygen is needed which results in more breaths and to get more breaths more blood is need to circulate which finally results in more work for the heart.

Also in my experience, thoughts of anxiety are more associated with chest breathing as compared to deep abdominal / diaphragmatic breathing.

So the simple analysis is, *if you want your heart to do less work, chest breathing or thoracic breathing is not the good option.*

Paradoxical Breathing

This type of breathing pattern involves combination of expanding the chest and contracting the abdominal muscles during inhalation process. In this breathing although the chest wall expands and lung volume is increased however the diaphragm simultaneously rises and reduces the gain of increase lung volume. This breathing pattern is called paradoxical breathing because the abdominal wall moves in rather than out during inhalation and out rather than in during exhalation process.

I am surprised to see many times in my yoga classes beginners use this kind of breathing because of their habit. All I can say that this is not the efficient way to breathe.

Deep abdominal breathing or **diaphragmatic breathing** is the best among all the breathing patterns. In this breathing exercise during inhalation the diaphragm moves downward, which pushes abdominal down and outward and during exhalation the diaphragm moves upward and abdomen moves inward. In this type of breathing we extract more energy from breath as compared to other two types of breath and it is the most natural and efficient way to breathe. Diaphragmatic breathing can be practiced either in standing position or sitting position or even in lying position on your back.

In my experience, if you can practice consciously slow and deep diaphragmatic breathing every day, you can feel the noticeable changes in your state of mind and certainly you can find the freedom from anxiety, stress and hypertension.

Why abdominal breathing (diaphragmatic breathing) is the most natural and efficient way to breathe?

There are many reasons for using the Diaphragmatic Breathing:

The lungs are pear shaped, with the narrow end pointing upwards. This means that with chest breathing, only the narrow top part of the lungs are used, rather than the larger deeper recesses accessed during diaphragmatic breathing. In Diaphragmatic breathing expansion is focused on lower area of lungs (more blood in lower area of lung because of gravity) where oxygen exchange can take place more efficiently with blood.

With each diaphragmatic breath the abdominal organs are massaged, they are stimulated and invigorated. This alternating squeezing and relaxing action helps to pump the blood through the organs of the abdomen and helps in moving waste through the intestines.

Less energy is required to breathe with the diaphragm muscle than with the chest muscles. Shallow chest breathing never empties the waste products from the deep recesses of your lungs where they accumulate and stagnate. Whenever possible breathe diaphragmatically.

Yogic Breath

Deep breathing exercise is recommended in day to day life as healthy breathing however, none of the above breathing patterns are complete. A complete breathing process is full yogic breath which combines three breathing exercises (abdominal, chest & clavicular) and everyday practice of full yogic breath in addition to slow and deep abdominal breath certainly helps in reducing stress and depression and helps in relaxation.

A full yogic breath begins with deep abdominal breathing and continuing the inhalation process through the rib cage and shoulder area. This breathing helps the person to store abundant energy within the body and you can work for the whole day and still experience by the end of the day that you are full of energy.

The yogic breathing can be performed everyday for short time as breathing exercise.

Why the speech of CEO & leaders is thrilling?

Have you ever wondered, why the speech of one speaker may thrill the audience, while the speech of another may have very little or no effect even though the second may speak in style.

The difference is the speech of the first speaker is charged with high energy. All the famous leaders you may find in history and present time have wonderful high energy level and when they speak people feel thrilled and people find them inspiring.

Full yogic breathing helps in increasing vitality and your energy level. Anyone with regular practice can start seeing the result within 4 to 6 week time. The important thing is right practice and consistency. The ill effect of tension and depression can be overcome or to a great extent reduced by this breathing technique.

Lifestyle, Body Energy level and Breath

The flow of energy in your body is affected by your lifestyle such as physical activities, work, sleep, food and sex. Your emotions, imagination or the thoughts can affect the energy of your body even more. Stress also depletes the energy flow and you may experience being totally drained of energy.

The breath is the most vital process of your body. If a person is engaged in deep thinking, relaxation or meditation, the breathing will be slow and steady. If the person is affected by negative emotions, the breathing will become fast, unsteady and irregular. The slow and deep breathing is very important for increasing the human life span!

If you observe the animals life span, you can notice that the animals with slow breath rate (elephants, tortoises, pythons) have a longer life span than the one with a fast breathing rate (dogs, rabbits) which live only for few years.

A slow breathing rate keeps the heart stronger and better nourished and leads to a longer life. By slow and deep breathing we increase the absorption of energy, enhancing our vitality and general wellbeing.

Part 2:

Practical Breathing Techniques

When the body and mind are constantly overworked their natural efficiency decreases. A few moments of stress i.e. anger, anxiety or irritation can consume great amount of energy leaving the person drained in their day to day life.

Psychosomatic illnesses such as diabetes, hypertension, migraine, etc arises from stress. If the mind is tense the stomach will also be tense and if the stomach is tense, the circulatory system is also tense.

However, if we are able to reduce our stress level, we can avoid most of the present day life style disease and can enjoy our healthy body and mind.

Have you ever noticed that from time to time after long hours of sleep you wake up feeling exhausted and you wonder why? The answer is simple: unless you are free from stress, your body and mind will always be tense and you can never feel relaxed.

However the good news is we can come out of stress at our own will and our body and mind can be reenergized by the simple breathing exercises.

Before going for practicing breathing exercises it is important to consider the following notes / precautions.

Notes for the practitioners of breathing exercise:

Breathing through nose or mouth: Always breathe through the nose with the awareness (unless specified by mouth). *Remember a simple concept that by nature, mouth is for eating and nose is for breathing.* Please do not try to reverse the nature functions. As you breathe in, know that you are breathing in. As you breathe out, know that you are breathing out. This will greatly enhance your general health and well-being.

Just for the enlightment nose performs not only the breathing function but it filters the air, moisturise the air, warms the air, it can smell, it secretes the mucus and performs many more functions etc. Now think for a moment if the mouth can perform all these functions………………………………….…………………..

Yes you are thinking correctly, mouth cannot perform all these functions, so please do not breathe through mouth unless specified in some special exercises.

Time of breathing practices: Simple slow and deep breathing exercise (Technique no 1) can be done any time,

However kapalabhati and Alternate Nostril breathing exercises can be done early in the morning for best results or just after sunset. Please remember to breathe in and out slowly and without a hurry in technique no 1, 2, 4 and 5.

Place of practice: It is good to practice in a room which is well ventilated. Please do not practice under a fan or direct sunlight.

Sitting Posture: Any comfortable sitting position is ok. The main point is body needs to be relaxed and back straight. Do not slump and do not lean forward. It is good to sit on folded blanket or cloth which is made from natural fibre.

Empty stomach: When practice kapalabhati and alternate nostril breathing exercise please make sure that your stomach is empty, i.e. your last meal should be around 3 and half hour before.

Straining while holding the breath: I have seen many time participants try to stain themselves particularly when holding the breath so that they can advance further.

I repeat again that please never strain your lungs while holding the breath when doing the practice of alternate nostril breathing exercise as lungs are delicate organs and forcefully holding the breath beyond your comfort level would only injure your lungs.

Some Symptoms:

Sometimes it does happen that when you start regular practice of alternate nostril exercise with breath retention, (technique no 5) you may experience constipation. If this happens to you please check yourself whether you drink plenty of water (8 to 10 glasses) or not.

If drinking less water please remember to drink enough water.

Breath retention and kapalabhati exercise should not be practice when you are ill.

Breath is life in itself and each incoming-breath brings the gift of life, and each out-flowing breath can be a natural release of tension and negativity.

Breathing Technique no 1

Diaphragmatic Breathing

Deep abdominal breathing or diaphragmatic breathing happens because of action of diaphragm. In this breathing exercise during inhalation, the diaphragm moves downward, which pushes abdominal down and outward and during exhalation the diaphragm moves upward and abdomen moves inward.

Abdominal breathing is the most natural and efficient breathing. One can observe a little baby breath since the moment of his/her birth and it is diaphragmatic breathing only.

For performing or learning abdominal breathing
First lie down flat on your back and relax your whole body. Check yourself if there is any tension in any of your body parts and if you find any tightness just release it. Now take your awareness towards your breath.

Next observe your natural breath and make sure you are not controlling it but only observing it.

Now place your left hand on the abdomen on your navel area.

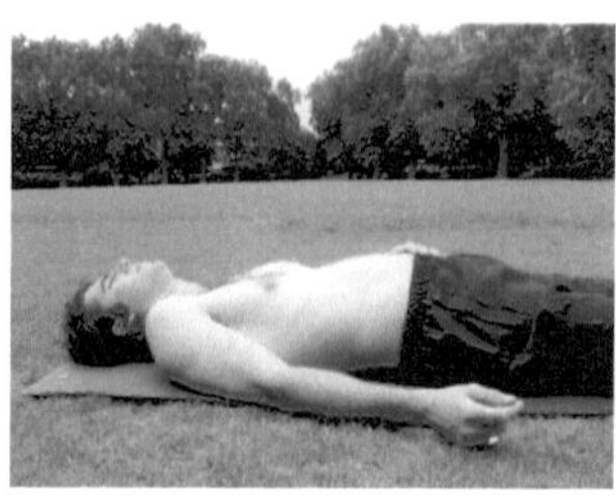

(Position of abdomen during inhalation)

If you are breathing naturally through your abdomen, your left hand (which is above abdomen) would move up with inhalation and down with exhalation.

Try to take your breath deeper and deeper into the lungs so that you feel the abdomen lifting as you breathe in and falling as you breathe out.

Gradually, you would notice that the abdomen is moving more firmly, and the chest moving less. As abdominal breathing becomes easier to you, try to let your breathing become *slower, deeper* and *smoother*.

The slow, deep and smooth breath would bring relaxation to the body and mind. This is the breathing pattern you can use all the times, while at rest or at work. Practice it until it becomes natural and unconscious.

Cautions:
Make sure that there are no jerks in flow of your breath. The flow of your breath should be smooth and without any noise.

Technique no 2

Full yogic breath

Full yogic breath combines the three breathing techniques. In yogic breath inhalation happens in three stages however in smooth way i.e. it looks as if single attempt to breathe in without jerk. It is better if this technique could be learnt first in presence of a qualified yoga trainer and later on can be practice on its own.

This type of breathing is very helpful in calming the nervous system and releasing stress.

Yogic breath technique step by step:

You can sit in a comfortable posture or you may lie down in relaxation posture called savasana, whichever position you prefer.

Observe your breath just outside your nostril area for next couple of breaths, say about 10 breaths.

Now inhale slowly and deeply (abdominal breathing) and when you feel that abdomen has comfortably expanded enough

then try expending chest area by expanding ribs and after ribs are expended comfortably, try inhaling little more air to expand upper portion of lungs and base of neck. In this process shoulders and collar bones would also move up a little.

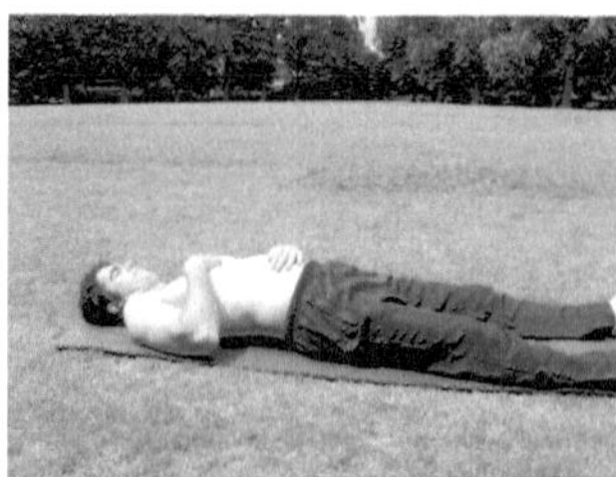

Now start to exhale slowly, relaxing lower neck and upper chest area, then chest and finally abdomen would be coming in. Try to exhale completely by pulling abdominal muscle in within your comfort level.

One inhalation and one exhalation is equal to one breath or one round of yogic breath. One can practice 10 rounds every day.

Cautions:
Make sure that there are no jerks in flow of your breath. The flow of your breath should be smooth and without any noise.

Technique no 3

Kapalabhati exercise

(Cleansing Breathing Exercise)

Kapala in Sanskrit means SKULL and Bhati means SHINING. Practicing kapalabhati on regular basis leads to shining skull and face with good health.

Kapalabhati is highly energizing abdominal breathing exercise. It cleans the respiratory passage and stimulates digestive organs.

Beginners can begin this exercise in mild form i.e. do not push your abdomen too much while exhaling.

What we do in Kapalbhati

In Kapalabhati we do quick exhalation and natural inhalation. Normally exhalation takes one fourth of the time of inhalation.

Quick exhalation and natural inhalation follow each other. This cycle of quick exhalation and natural inhalation is repeated several times.

How to do Kapalabhati

Step 1) Sit in a comfortable crossed leg position with back straight. Hands comfortably resting on knees. Face to be relaxed.

Step 2) Inhale deeply through both nostrils, expanding Abdomen.

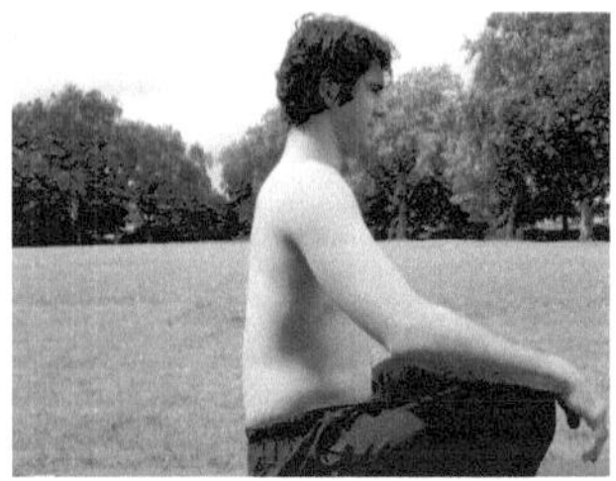

Step 3) Now exhale with the forceful contraction of abdominal muscles. (*Pull the abdomen in by quickly contracting the abdominal muscles and exhale through the nose*).

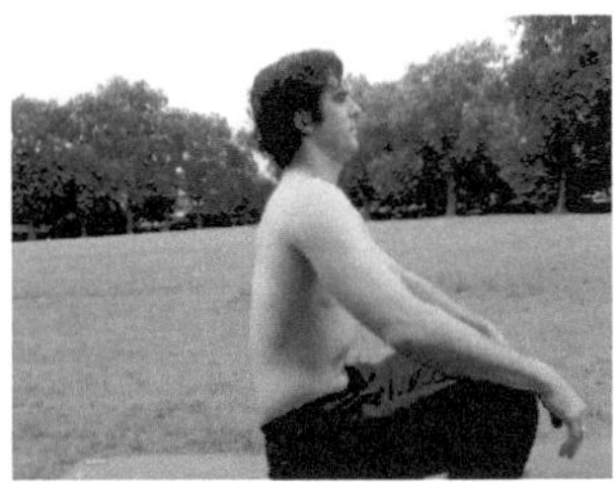

Model Duncan Hogg

The air is pushed out of lungs by contraction of the diaphragm.

Step 4) After exhalation you inhale again but inhalation should not involve any effort.

To inhale just relax and the lungs will automatically expand and fill with air. One can begin with 10 respirations. After completing 10 quick exhalations and natural inhalations relax and breathe naturally. This is one round. One can start the practice of Kapalabhati with 3 rounds.

Benefits of Kapalabhati

1) Kapalabhati cleanses the lungs and entire respiratory system.

2) The blood is purified and body gets an increased supply of oxygen to all cells.
3) Digestion is improved.
4) Abdominal muscles are strengthened.
5) Prepares the mind for meditation.
6) Energises the mind for mental work.

Precautions:

Kapalabhati should not be practice by those suffering from

a) Heart disease
b) High blood pressure
c) Hernia
d) Vertigo

e) When Asthmatic attack in progress.

f) If pain or dizziness is experienced (*it is preferable to stop the practice till the sensation has passed. Practice can be restarted with less force*).

g) Quick exhalation should be comfortable to oneself, i.e. *quick exhalation should not be too forceful.*

h) In case of pregnancy Kapalabhati should not be done.

Common Mistakes:

1) Abdomen is contracted while inhaling. *This mistake is done most often by people who are habitual of breathing mostly through chest or paradoxical breathing.*

2) Shoulders are contracted to push the air out when exhaling.

3) Back and shoulders move during exercise.

Point to Note:

a) Exercise should not be done if you are feeling uncomfortable at any time anywhere in the body during the exercise.

b) Rapid breathing used in this technique should be from the *abdomen* and not from the chest.

c) Kapalabhati should be practice on an *empty stomach* only.

d) Ideally when doing this exercise along with yoga and meditation, Kapalabhati should be practiced after the yoga postures and relaxation (*at least 10 minutes*) and before meditation.

e) *People with poor lungs capacity should be very careful* while doing this exercise and please do not exhale forcefully.

f) Chest should not move very much.

g) *I recommend that in the beginning one should learn this exercise with yoga teacher only.*

"Emotional and mental state of person are difficult to control, however they are linked with breath and breath can be controlled i.e. emotional and mental state of human being can be controlled by controlling breath"

Technique no 4:

Alternate Nostril Breathing

(<u>Without</u> breath retention)

A normal person breathe predominantly through one nostril at a time i.e. either through right nostril or left nostril and flow of breath changes every 2 to 3 hours from one nostril to another.

Left hemisphere of the brain controls the right side of body and predominantly involved with logical thinking, analysis and mathematical functions. So when right nostril is clear and freely flowing, in that case right side of body is predominant (and left hemisphere of brain).

The right hemisphere of brain controls left part of body and is involved in more creative and artistic functions. And when left nostril is clear, in this case left part of body is dominant (and right hemisphere of brain).

Also the point to note is, if one nostril remains open for several hours without changing the flow to other nostril this is a sign of some imbalance and if only one nostril remains active or predominant throughout the day i.e. 24 hours this is a sign that illness may pursue or already in progress.

Simple alternate nostril breathing exercise helps to establish the natural rhythm of breath and regular practice helps human being in attaining healthy physical and mental state.

Any disease in body is a sign of imbalance in body's energy level and this simple *alternate nostril breathing exercise brings balance in the body energy level and helps the body to remain disease free* along with calmness.

Also Alternate Nostril Breathing (*Without breath retention*) purifies the energy channels in the body which carries the increased energy to some areas of the brain.

It is very important that the channels be purified first to cope with the increased energy created by advance breathing exercise of breath retention.

It is preferable to close your eyes during practice of alternate nostril breathing.

How to do Alternate Nostril Breathing: (*Without breath retention*)

1. Inhale completely through the left nostril, keeping the right nostril closed with the right thumb. This can be done by counting up to "4" mentally.

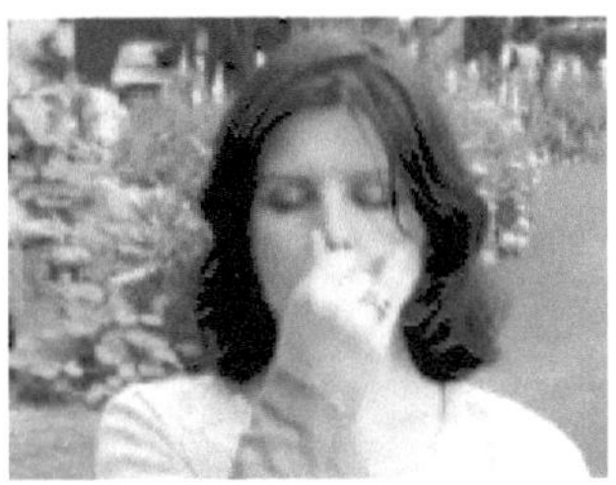

2. Release the right nostril and exhale completely to a count of "4", counting mentally (Close left nostril).

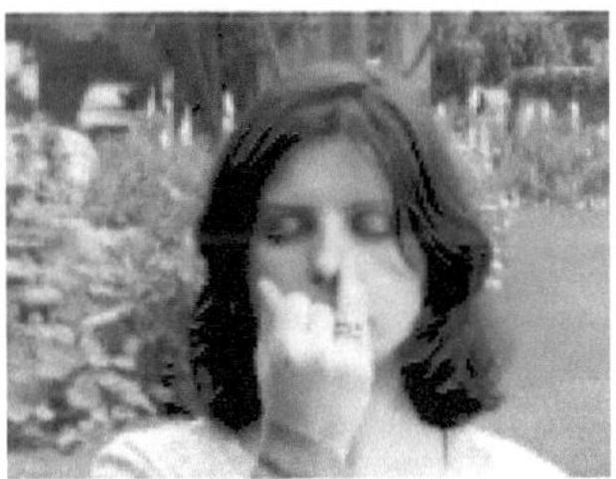

3. Inhale fully through the right nostril to a count of "4". (Left nostril closed).

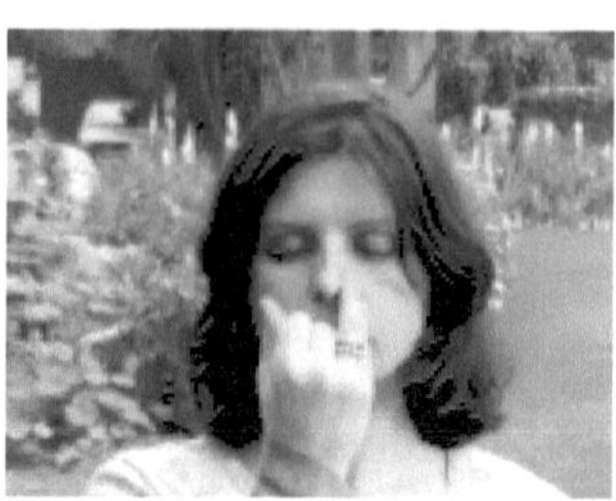

4. Release the left nostril and exhale completely to a count of "4" (Right nostril closed).

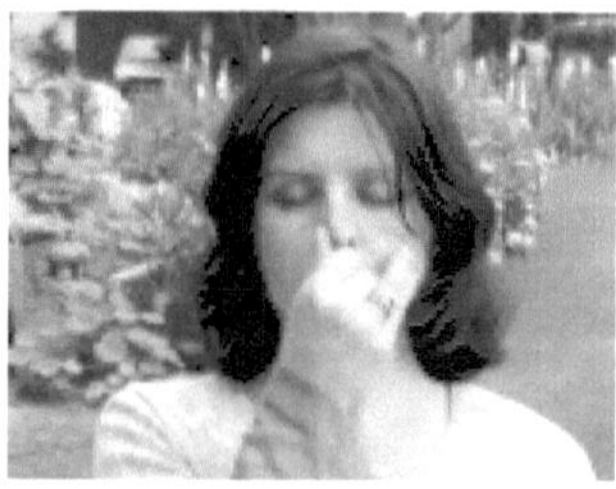

This is one round. At least 20 rounds should be practiced daily and gradually increased to 40 rounds.

Next step after you master this ratio:

After 8 to 12 weeks of regular practice depending upon your comfort level, the "count" of the exercise may be increased.

For example, inhaling to the count of 5 and then exhaling to the count of 5.

After completing this breathing exercise it is good to relax for about 5 to 10 minutes.

By nature

"Mouth is for eating

And

Nose is for breathing"

Technique no 5

Alternate Nostril Breathing

(With breath retention)

This is advance breathing exercise and should be done ***only*** under the guidance of experienced yoga trainer.

Sit in any comfortable position. You can sit in any position in which you are comfortable and can sit for about 10 – 15 minutes without any pain.

You also have the option to sit on chair which has straight back or may sit with the support of wall in case if you cannot sit with back straight.

The main point is comfortable position and straight back with relax body. Observe the breath for about 2 min or say about 25 -30 breaths.

Preparing for Alternate Nostril Breathing exercise (with breath retention)

Raise the right hand. Make the Vishnu Mudra by folding down the index and middle fingers as shown below.

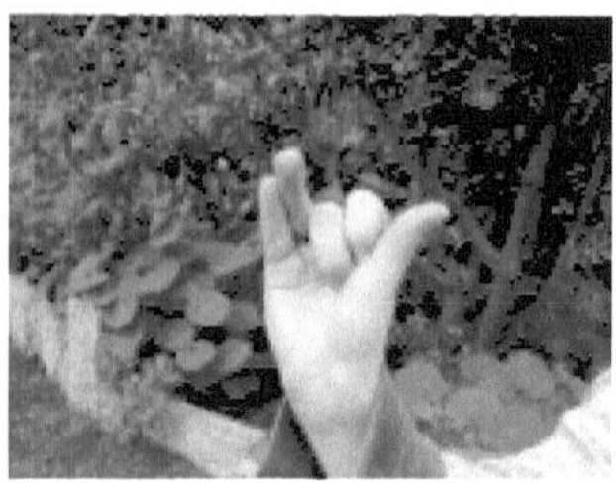

How to do Alternate Nostril Breathing:

1. Inhale completely through the left nostril, keeping the right nostril closed with the right thumb (as shown in picture below). This can be done by counting up to "4" mentally.

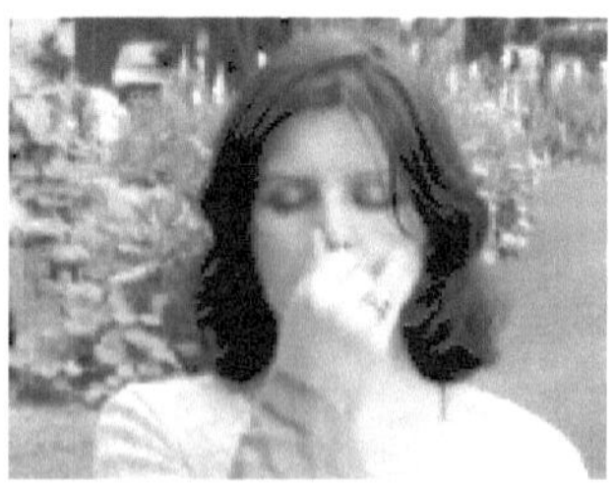

2. Close the left nostril with the two end fingers so that both nostrils are closed (as shown in picture below). Retain the breath to a count of "4" counting mentally.

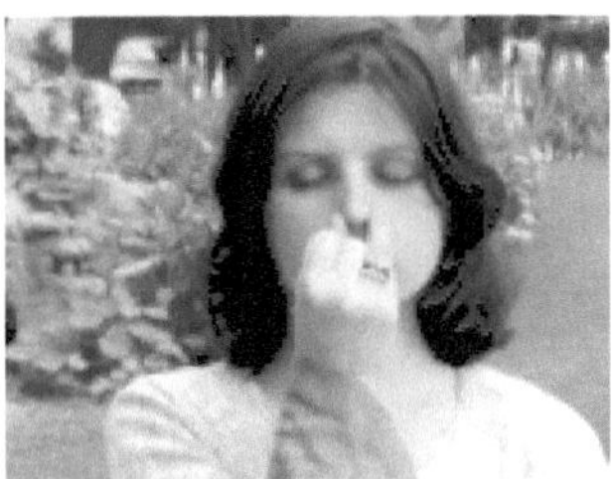

3. Release the right nostril and exhale completely to a count of "4", counting mentally as shown in picture below.

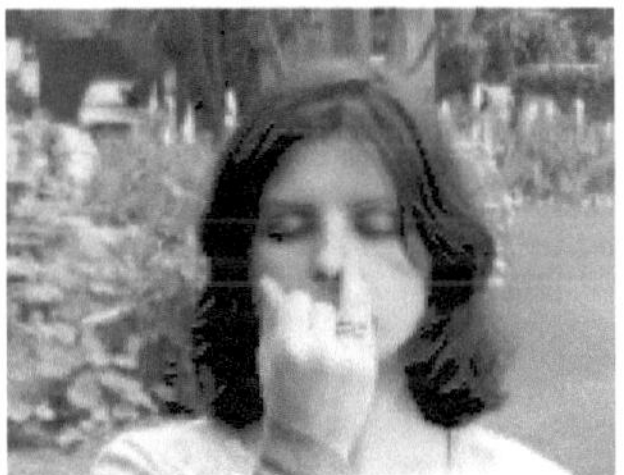

4. Inhale fully through the right nostril to a count of "4" (as shown in picture below).

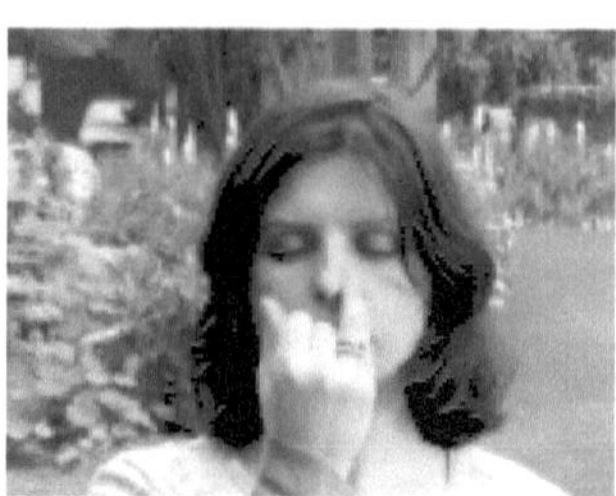

5. Both nostrils closed and retain the breath to a count of "4".

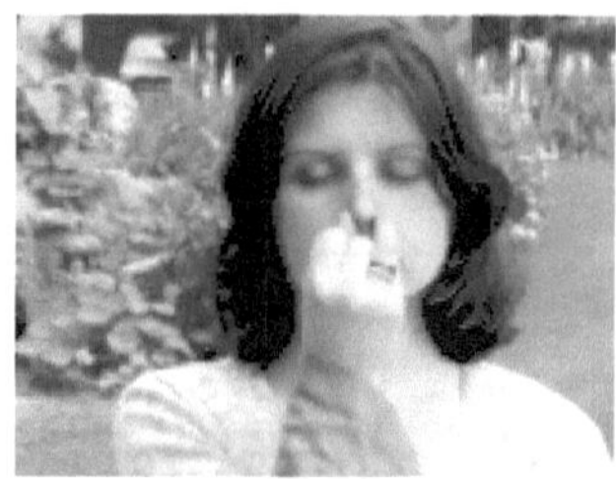

6. Release the left nostril and exhale completely to a count of "4" as shown in picture below.

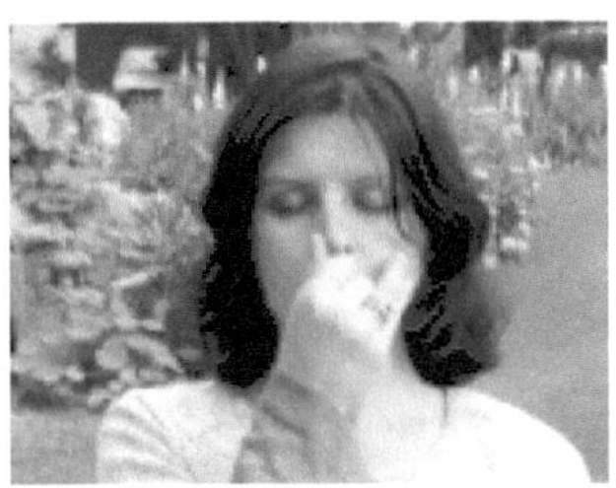

This is one round.
At least 10 rounds should be practiced daily.

Next step

After 8 to 12 weeks of regular practice depending upon your comfort level the "count" of the exercise may be increased.

For example it can be inhaling to the count of 5, then retaining the breath to the count of 5 and then releasing the breath to the count of 5.

Next step:

After you master this ratio of 1:1:1 (i.e. inhaling the breath to the count of 5, retaining breath to the count of 5 and exhaling the breath to the count of 5,) one can increase the ratio to 1:1:2 (Inhaling to the count of 5, retaining the breath to the count of 5 and exhaling the breath to the count of 10).

Next Step:
After mastering the ratio of 1:1:2 increase the ratio to 1:2:2. (Inhale the breath to the count of 5, retain the breath to the count of 10 and exhale to the count of 10).

Next Step:
After mastering the ratio of 1:2:2 increase this ratio to 1:3:2 and finally 1:4:2.

Once you reach to the ratio of 1:4:2 then stick to this ratio. For example: you inhale for 4 seconds; you retain the breath for 16 seconds and exhale for 8 seconds , never change the ratio. You may also increase the number of rounds of Alternate nostril breathing.

Benefits of Alternate Nostril Breathing:
Physical benefits

1. Alternate Nostril Breathing cleanses and strengthens the lungs and entire respiratory system.

2. During retention, there is the highest rate of gaseous exchange in the lungs. Because of the increase in the pressure, more oxygen goes from the lungs into the blood and more CO2 and other waste products pass from the blood into the lungs for elimination during exhalation.

3. As exhalation is twice the time of inhalation, stale air and waste products are drained from the lugs.

4. This breathing exercise is good for people who are suffering from low blood pressure.

Mental Psychic benefits:

1. Alternate Nostril Breathing helps to calm the mind, making it lucid and steady.

2. It makes the body light and the eyes shiny.

Common Mistakes:

1. Back is not straight.
2. The breath is not smooth.

Precautions:

(1) I would like to repeat here, *it is strongly advised that this exercise should be learnt from an experienced yoga teacher only* and not on your own or by watching TV channels or DVD.

(2) ***Beginners*** should not try this exercise of breath retention rather they can try simple Alternate Nostril Breathing ***without*** breath retention.

(3)Please do not try to hold breath beyond your comfort level as it will not benefit you rather can hurt you as lungs are delicate organs.

(4) People who are suffering from eye or ear problem (like glaucoma or pus in the ear) can be more cautious and preferably do not hold breath.

(5) Please make sure that during practice of breath retention, you should not feel any strain in eyes, ears, thighs and arms.

If you are beginner you can observe that quite often we have tendency to tense our arm.

(6) The place for breathing exercises should be well ventilated.

(7) If you are suffering from high blood pressure or heart trouble, you may please avoid holding the breath.

Stress Monitor

Before beginning breathing exercise plan, please take couple of minutes to fill in the following stress monitor.

	Stress Monitor	
S.N.	Indicators	Before Beginning
1	Blood Pressure (High)	
	(Low)	
2	Hours of sleep (average per week)	
3	Quality of sleep (1 to 5) (1 lowest and 5 the best, average for the week)	
4	Stress level (1 to 5) (1 lowest and 5 highest, average for the week)	
5	Overall energy level (1 to 5) (1 lowest and 5 highest)	

Practice Record

Starting Date……………………………………..

	Week 1	Sun	Mon	Tue	Wed	Thu	Fri	Sat
S.N	Breathing Technique							
1	Simple slow &Deep Abdominal Breathing							
2	Full Yogic Breath							
3	Kapalabhati							
4	Alternate Nostril Breathing (without breath retention)							

After week 1 please record below, how do you feel / improvement

Practice Record

	Week 2	Sun	Mon	Tue	Wed	Thu	Fri	Sat
S.N	Breathing Technique							
1	Simple slow &Deep Abdominal Breathing							
2	Full Yogic Breath							
3	Kapalabhati							
4	Alternate Nostril Breathing (without breath retention)							

After week 2 please record below, how do you feel / improvement

Practice Record

	Week 3	Sun	Mon	Tue	Wed	Thu	Fri	Sat
S.N	Breathing Technique							
1	Simple slow &Deep Abdominal Breathing							
2	Full Yogic Breath							
3	Kapalabhati							
4	Alternate Nostril Breathing (without breath retention)							

After week 3 please record below, how do you feel / improvement

Practice Record

	Week 4	Sun	Mon	Tue	Wed	Thu	Fri	Sat
S.N	Breathing Technique							
1	Simple slow &Deep Abdominal Breathing							
2	Full Yogic Breath							
3	Kapalabhati							
4	Alternate Nostril Breathing (without breath retention)							

After week 4 please record below, how do you feel / improvement

Stress Monitor

After 4 weeks of regular practice of breathing exercise, please take couple of minutes to fill in the following stress monitor.

	Stress Monitor	
S.N.	Indicators	After 4 week
1	Blood Pressure (High)	
	(Low)	
2	Hours of sleep (average per week)	
3	Quality of sleep (1 to 5) (1 lowest and 5 the best, average for the week)	
4	Stress level (1 to 5) (1 lowest and 5 highest, average for the week)	
5	Overall energy level (1 to 5) (1 lowest and 5 highest)	

Dear practitioner,

Please note that you can begin with only the first 2 breathing exercises initially and later on you can incorporate exercise number third and fourth in your schedule, if your time permits.

Breathing exercise number five is more for information purpose and should only be tried after couple of months of practicing exercise number four and that too under the guidance of an experienced teacher.

While practicing breathing exercises if you come across any question, you are welcome to send me your query at: Email: info@subodhgupta.com

More information about us is available at www.subodhgupta.com

I wish you good health and happiness in your life.

With Best Regards
Subodh Gupta

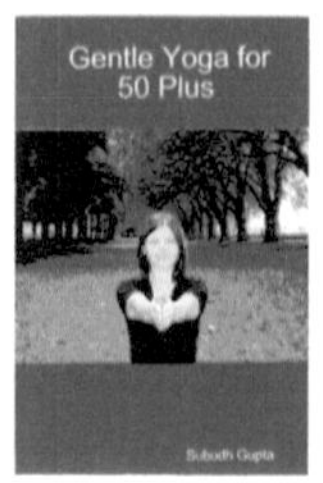

Gentle Yoga for 50 Plus

"A perfect gift of health for your parents"

The only book on Gentle Yoga for people in the age group of 50 plus. The exercises explained in this book are also beneficial if suffering from arthritis or rheumatism.

Paperback/ £5.95/ 68 pages

7 Food Habits for Weight Loss *Forever*

Stay Healthy and Slim *Forever*

"For anybody who wants to lose weight and gain health forever"

"Managing perfect body weight is not a complicated rocket science. Our body is made up of food which we eat during our day to day life. If we are overweight or obese at the moment then one thing is certain that the food which we eat is not good."

Healthy Food Habits = Good Health + Perfect Body Weight *Forever*

ISBN 978-0-9556882-0-1
Page 68 / Soft Cover / £4.95

All our books are available at Amazon.com, Barnes and Nobles

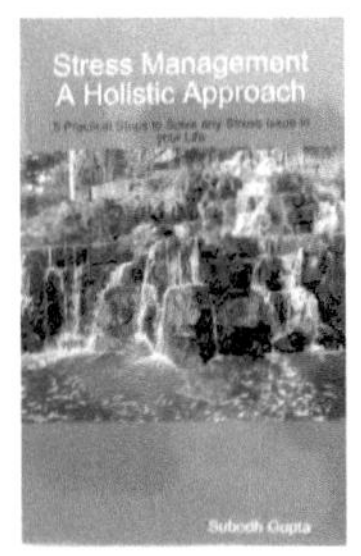

Stress Management a Holistic Approach

5 Steps plan to manage any Stress issue in your life

Many illnesses such as diabetes, migraine, asthma, ulcer and even cancer arise because of excessive Stress over the period of time.

You may have any kind of problem or issue in your life, once you follow the 5 steps described in this book you are on your way to Stress free life. If there is a problem then there has to be a solution and this book is all about solution.

ISBN 978-0-9556882-1-8
Page 80 / Soft Cover / £4.95

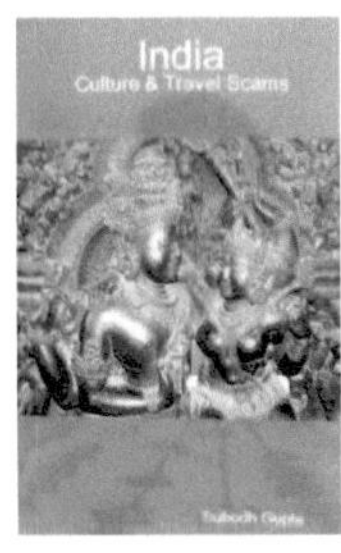

India Culture and Travel scams

"The only book on travel scams targeted at western tourists in India"

This is a practical book about understanding Indian culture and travel scams in India and is based on real life experiences.

This book will help you to avoid embarrassing mistakes and prepare you to feel confident in unfamiliar situations.

Content in this book includes Indian social customs, their perception about Western women, their religion, what motivates them, travel scams targeted at Western tourists and of course what not to discuss with Indians, etc.

Page 112/Paper Back / £5.95
ISBN 978-0-9556882-6-3

www.ingramcontent.com/pod-product-compliance
Ingram Content Group UK Ltd.
Pitfield, Milton Keynes, MK11 3LW, UK
UKHW041837200726
13854UKWH00003BA/1179